I0455472

WHAT ABOUT GOD?

Healthy Weight Loss
through
Commitment, Meditation, and Prayer

This book is dedicated to my parents, Harles and Jean. They did the best they could with what they had. I thank God for them!

A Special Thank You To:

Barbara, Creflo, Eddie, Joel, Joyce, and T.D.

You present God in a way that I could not help but love him!

II Corinthians 5:14-21

Our firm decision is to work from this focused center: One man died for everyone. That puts everyone in the same boat. He included everyone in his death so that everyone could also be included in his life, a resurrection life, a far better life than people ever lived on their own.

Because of this decision we don't evaluate people by what they have or how they look. We looked at the Messiah that way once and got it all wrong, as you know. We certainly don't look at him that way anymore. Now we look inside, and what we see is that anyone united with the Messiah gets a fresh start, is created new. The old life is gone; a new life burgeons! Look at it! All this comes from the God who settled the relationship between us and him, and then called us to settle our relationships with each other.

God put the world square with himself through the Messiah, giving the world a fresh start by offering forgiveness of sins. God has given us the task of telling everyone what he is doing. We're Christ's representatives. God uses us to persuade men and women to drop their differences and enter into God's work of making things right between them. We're speaking for Christ himself now; Become friends with God, he's already a friend with you. How? You ask. In Christ. God put the wrong on him who never did anything wrong so we could be put right with God.

Table of Contents

Introduction
How This Book Helps

Most overweight people are full of excuses for their condition. The people I interviewed while researching this book all had some type of physical, nutritional, or health-related issue that prevents them from working out (so they say; don't laugh—it really is not funny). I heard so many excuses that the thought of writing a book titled *101 Excuses for Being Fat* crossed my mind (several times). It is really sad because these people, like many others, are missing out on the beautiful life God has planned for them. Because of the limitations they have set by making 101 excuses, being obese, or being overweight, God's plan will not be implemented according to his will. It amazes me that a determination to eat what you want when you want and praying for a good piece of cake cannot be exchanged for praying to have a healthy heart, a healthy weight, or low cholesterol. While interviewing these people, I realized how much of their problem is an inside job, because I saw their pain. Some had blocked it out so much that they did not realize it still existed. Working from the inside out through God and Jesus Christ had not crossed their minds. Sure, some were full of godly sayings, quotes from the Bible, and prayers; however, I saw no attempt to apply Christian precepts to their weight problems at all.

How can a Christian say "I just can't lose this weight" when we believe that God is all powerful, all knowing, and in all places? When you worship, do you really believe, or are you just saying that you do? If this is a reality, then why not call on God to relieve the pain that has caused your current condition? Why do so many people choose to believe God cannot help with the weight problem? And honesty is needed: the problem really isn't the weight— you are. Why are you the problem? You are the problem because you do not believe in God as much as you think you do. If you did, then you would not try so many diets, excuses, quick fixes, or eating to fix your pain. Believing in and trusting God is what matters. If you truly have faith, then everything you place before God will turn out just the way it is supposed to in all cases. God does not want us to suffer because we do not stand firm in our faith.

This book is designed to give you insight into what you already have—knowledge of how powerful God is and how Jesus is the truth, the light and the way. We no longer have to feel ashamed nor do we have to hide behind food. There is hope if you believe it. The relationship you have with Jesus strengthens the one you have with God the Father. To get to the Father, you have to know Jesus. The temple you live in was provided by God; therefore, it is up to you to take care of it. God loves us as we are. However, God wants us to love ourselves and our neighbors. Question: If you saw people treating themselves the way you treat yourself, what would you say? What would you do? Be that person that you know needs help and go to God through Jesus to conquer the problem with a suitable solution. Be an example of the power of God by showing others what can be done through Jesus. I am not talking about a skinny solution; this is about a healthy one. If your weight is fine and you need to tone, this book is for you. If your health is not very good and your weight is a little off, then this book is for you. If you need to stop dieting, get on a path of healthy living, and place your cares on God, this book is for you. The only medication we need is God's love. The greatest gift of all is love; love yourself enough to give yourself to God!

Chapter 1

Why I Wrote This Book

As a child I experienced emotional and sexual abuse. In my environment everyone had self-esteem issues. Food became my friend. I ate food to make myself feel different. I ate food to make everything peaceful and acceptable for the moment. I ate food to feel pleasure in life. I ate food to know that life was worth living. I ate food to gain courage for the next moment, hour or day. I really looked forward to eating something that would take the unpleasant feelings away so I could make it through the day. I believed, with all my heart and mind that I was alone and that I had no one to protect or care about me. I always felt like I was holding my breath until someone gave approval for my existence. I wondered how this God that everyone talked about could let me live in such horrible fear. After several years, as my self-esteem sank lower and lower and I was dieting, using pills, and trying other methods to lose weight (anything but God), I got extremely depressed and gave up.

At one time in my life, I did not believe in religion, in God, or in Jesus Christ. I thought it was all a lie. I reflected on the way I was treated, the fears and feelings that surfaced daily and haunted me. If there were a God or if Jesus were real, how could they let all of this happen to me? I did not have any role models, nor were there people near me to prove anything different to me. After I had lived many years of a self-willed life, people who were positive examples of God's will showed up (I know God sent them), and I began reading the Bible.

I started reading the New Testament and learned how Jesus died for us and that God loves us as we are. I wasn't really interested in religion, but I wanted to know how to get rid of the pain in my life. I wanted to learn how to stop pleasing people and how to love myself.

Once I learned about spirituality, about God, and about Jesus Christ, I began to see how I had blocked all that God wanted to offer me. I learned (and am still learning) that I will always make mistakes and will not be perfect, but that Jesus died so that I could live. Jesus gave his life for my sins; all I have to do is ask for forgiveness and live by God's word in the Bible. Through God and Jesus Christ, I also learned that many of my problems were of my own design and delivery. The abuse I had experienced as a child wasn't happening to me any more, and I didn't have to live with it.

I learned that food never really worked; I just believed it did. In fact, it made me feel worse because I continued to go up and down with my weight. When I gained weight, my self-esteem would plummet. I depended on others to tell me how I should feel. I never saw the beauty that was inside; I felt ugly, and that is what I saw on the outside. No matter how much I weighed, I never gave myself approval. I also found out that I did not like nor love myself. I was my worst critic. I could no longer blame God nor anyone else; I had to find out how I could learn to love and like myself as I was, so that becoming new would be done with ease, peace, and love.

I also had to learn to be obedient to God and to be of service to others. Because I have choices, what I do and how I live begins and ends with me. God is always there for me, even when it feels that God is not. Today, I choose to learn how to allow God to lead my life. Taking care of my temple—my body, the house I live in—is being grateful to God for giving it to me. It also allows me to acknowledge God's power and to be an example of it. I know God loves me. I look at what Jesus did for us, and I ask myself, "How can you continue to live as if God does not exist?" Jesus gave us a way; we just have to accept and live by it.

Most people worship or believe in God or a Higher Power. If this is true, then why do so many people turn to outside help, such as humans, to meet weight-loss goals? Many practice their belief or religion with intense fervor; but when it comes to using that passion or power for their healing, the focus is not there. I am not saying that getting help from others to reach a goal weight or to live more healthily is out of the question. I am saying, however, that putting God and Jesus Christ first is the way to do this. Otherwise our efforts will not work; they will continue to be the temporary fix we have always received. In a nutshell, I believe that I am supposed to help people in whatever way I can. That is why I wrote this book and will write other books.

It is better to trust in the Lord than to put confidence in Man. *Psalm 118:8*

Chapter 2
What Experience Tells Us

Aaah! This scale cannot be correct! How did I get to this weight? Just two weeks ago I weighed 9 lbs less than I do now. Eight weeks ago I weighed 14 lbs less than I did last week. Last year at this time, I was 40 lbs lighter, and before that about 10 years ago, I weighed 50 lbs less than I did at the time this book was published.

I have fluctuated in losing and gaining weight constantly since I was a child. However, since 1999, I have been conscious of what has happened. It is now 2008, I am working on reaching a healthy weight, and I am eliminating and preventing any physical health issues. That means I have to work from the inside out, and God has to be in the center.

I used to try diets that promised a loss of 10 lbs in 4 days; I would declare that I would do it for one month to lose 40 1bs. That never worked! Then I would realize that I had done this before and had lost only 7 lbs because I could not stick to it at all. Afterwards, I would gain 5 1bs back within a week because I had been starving myself. As soon as I ate a piece of bread, the weight was pasted onto my hips. I really needed to map out a plan that worked for me. But God was nowhere in the picture.

Does any of this sound familiar to you? Have you gone through this cycle, said these things at any time during your life? My entire life has consisted of dieting and getting to the right size. How boring is that? My friends used to say that I had an "anorexic mentality" because no matter how much I weighed, in my opinion,

I always looked huge in the mirror. I always focused on what I thought other people thought about how I looked, and I wanted approval from them to say that I was pretty enough, slim enough, or good enough. I never, ever, not once asked God to help me: Never!

Experience tells us that dieting does not work. If dieting really did work, then new and improved plans would not continue to be developed. Experience also tells us that we have to diet all of the time instead of maintaining a healthy weight at all times. Why? Because we have not yet learned that achieving a healthy weight is really an inside job; we are always working on the outside. Diets work on the outside, not the inside. You have to get right on the inside, and then the outside will get what it needs, too. Get your spirit right through God and Jesus. Do you think that you were put on this earth to be totally consumed with dieting all of the time? How selfish is that? We are supposed to be helping someone else, serving God by helping other people!

What we know about our eating (other than that we eat to live) is that it is emotional. Our state of being is unacceptable to us, but we continue to live the way we are. We somehow think we have to be a size 2 when a healthy body, mind, and spirit would suffice. If your ankles are swollen all of the time or if you get tired after walking 20 feet, then you may need to address your weight issues. High cholesterol, diabetes, heart problems, kidney malfunction, liver deterioration, etc., can be attributed to excessive weight or inappropriate diets and not enough exercise. Go to God for the answer and pray for guidance and direction.

Our reliance upon God is to be used in all areas of our lives; however, we hardly rely on God for anything. We say that our reliance is upon God, but our actions show something totally different. I respect all religions and spiritual practices, as they have their purpose for those who choose to live by them. I, on the other hand, choose not to practice a religion, but rather simply to love God and Jesus Christ; knowing that Jesus died for my sins and that God loves me is enough for me. *Whatever you choose to practice,* <u>use it</u> to help you with solutions in all areas of your life.

Stop allowing the past to dictate your future. No one is responsible for your current state of being but YOU! Call on God's help to bring you into a state of health and wellness. Many people need counseling in addition to prayer and meditation. Certain deep issues should be resolved with professional help; God will guide you to this if it is necessary. Some people may just need prayer and meditation. Whatever works, use it! Stop mistreating yourself and missing out on the joyful life that was promised you. Come on, you cannot possibly tell me that you are content being on a diet all of the time. The focal point of your day is losing weight? How can you have time to do anything else or live the life promised to you if you constantly think about losing weight? Have you asked God to help? When and if you asked, did you believe that God was going to do it? If so, then why are you always dieting or feeling guilty about eating certain foods? Get real; come to believe in and rely on God to deliver

you from the bondage in which you currently
live.

Give your entire attention to what God is doing
right now, and don't get worked up about what
may or may not happen tomorrow. God will help
you deal with whatever hard things come up
when the time comes. *Matthew 6:34*

Chapter 3
Why We Diet

We diet because our lives lack discipline, because we have issues that are unresolved, because we have unreasonable expectations, because we have needs that are not being met, because we want to be someone that we are not, because we listen to the advertisements and eat food that is not good for us, and because we do not go to God through Jesus Christ to achieve a permanent solution.

We want a quick fix that can change us on the outside without making changes on the inside. If we do not have to look on the inside, we will not because the past hurts. That is why we diet—we never get to the core of the problem. We look at the temporary fix that is unrealistic and then think that all is well once we reach that goal. The point is, we keep reaching the same goal. Why not reach it once and for all by taking inventory, confessing all to God, and making amends to ourselves?

We diet because we lie to ourselves. We eat food that we know will put weight on us; then we lie and say that it will not hurt us. We continue to buy larger clothing sizes without looking at why we are gaining weight in the first place. Eating healthily does not cause you to gain weight. Unhealthy eating does cause weight gain and can produce other physical or psychological issues.

Exercise daily in God - no spiritual flabbiness, please! Workouts at the gymnasium are useful, but a disciplined life in God is far more so, making you fit both today and forever. You can count on this. Take it to heart. *Timothy 4:7-10*

Chapter 4

Dieting vs. Healthy Living

Some may attribute obesity and fluctuating weight gain to negative emotions or trauma. Because of our ability to tell ourselves everything but the truth, unhealthiness remains present. Many people neither love nor like themselves. Start loving God; then you will learn to love yourself as you are. When you learn to love yourself where you are, your life will change. How often have you said any of the following?

- Nobody loves me;
- I was born fat and will always be fat;
- I will start my eating plan tomorrow;
- Eating this will make me feel better;
- The trauma will go away eventually;
- I cannot leave him or her because I do not know what to do;

- I will eat one more piece of cake, then I will start my diet;
- I cannot lose weight, I have tried;
- I will just buy new clothes since I have gained weight;
- My weight is fine; I just gained a few pounds.

You get the picture, right? What we tell ourselves is our belief system. You have the power to change your belief system through God.

How often do you call on God to give you the strength and courage to lose weight and then BELIEVE that it will happen that the weight will stay off for good if you trust God and do the work? When you call on God, do you change your lifestyle to work for what you have asked? *Oh, I get it; the change will come without your lifting a finger? No!* It is good practice to continue to tell yourself what you cannot do, to look in the mirror and pretend that you do not see what is there, and to eat in an unhealthy manner because you cannot change, right? Wrong!

It is all an inside job. What I mean by this is that what you are on the inside shows on the outside. In other words, your lack of self esteem and your inability to trust and rely on God is why you are looking and feeling the way you do. I suggest you keep reading, channel your emotions into a determination to change, and God will make this possible. You have to be willing to change; it is not going to be as simple as buying that next piece of cake, but the change will feel better than if you eat that cake. On the following pages, there is no temporary fix—only a permanent one.

Read on! No matter what your religious or spiritual beliefs, this book will work for you. Have an open mind and remember that it is about changing your lifestyle and trusting in God, not trusting in People! God will put the people in your path to guide you to success. The problem is that <u>you</u> keep picking the people to help, and that is why your previous attempts to lose weight have not worked. Pick God instead; whatever you ask, have faith in God's works!

So be content with who you are, and don't put on airs. God's strong hand is on you, he'll promote you at the right time. Live carefree before God; he is most careful with you.
I Peter 5:6-7

Fear of Human Opinion Disables; Trust in God protects you from that. *Proverbs 29:25*

The first thing one must do when attempting a major life adjustment is to trust God. Too often there is interference from coveting or imaging ourselves after someone else. Trust that God has made *you* perfect. Your job is to find out who *you* are and not try to be like other people. We miss our blessings when the goal is to look and be like someone other than ourselves. Be yourself! If you really believe and trust in God, know that you are beautifully made and that you have every opportunity to experience just that! Stop basing who you are on what others may say you should be. The image you should strive to achieve is the one in the mirror, not the picture of someone else. What other people think is none of your business. Focus on honoring God by trusting that he made a beautiful person, and do not focus what you think others will think about you.

**

And therefore the Lord [earnestly] waits [expecting, looking, and longing] to be gracious to you; . . . For the Lord is a God of justice. Blessed (happy, fortunate, to be envied) are all those who [earnestly] wait for Him, who expect and look and long for Him [for His victory], His favor, His love, His peace, His joy, and His matchless, unbroken companionship.
Isaiah 30:18

Believe that God has more in store for you than a lifetime of dieting. Do you honestly believe that God wants you to spend day in and day out focusing on yourself? That is what dieting does; it consumes your thoughts with how bad or fat you look, obsession takes over, and the saga continues. God has an abundance of blessings in store for you. Take heed to

What About God?

who God is and to what he does for you. Enjoy who you are and live in accordance to the blessings and love of God.

**

God will provide rain for the seeds you sow. The grain that grows will be abundant. . . Better yet, on the Day God heals his people of the wounds and bruises from the time of punishment, moonlight will flare into sunlight, and sunlight, like a whole week of sunshine at once, will flood the land. *Isaiah 30:23-26*

Plant the seed to discover the real you. Once the seed is planted, know that God will provide an abundance of growth for you. What will be revealed is much greater than you can ever imagine. Stop living in the past, and come into the present with God. God will provide the healing you deserve for the pain you have suffered. Stop and give God the opportunity to allow you to live the life He has in store for you.

**

Be prepared. You're up against far more than you can handle on your own. Take all the help you can get, every weapon God has issued, so that when it's all over but the shouting you'll still be on your feet. Truth, righteousness, peace, faith, and salvation are more than words. Learn how to apply them. You'll need them throughout your life. God's Word is an indispensable weapon. In the same way, prayer is essential in this ongoing warfare. Pray hard and long. Pray for your brothers and sisters. Keep your eyes open. Keep each other's spirits up so that no one falls behind or drops out.
Ephesians 6:13-18

Apply God's word to your life to remain prepared. The road to success is full of trials and tribulations that can be overcome through God. Remember to pray for and gain support from others throughout the process. You are not alone; God is walking beside you and carrying you when you need it.

Chapter 6
Feelings

What we eat and when we eat have a lot to do with our feelings. Feelings are not facts, and they come and go. But God can be present in your life forever. Those who have experienced trauma as children might use food as a comfort throughout their lives. Those individuals will have to learn to replace food with prayers to God, journaling, and meditation. These practices may be harder for you than for others because of what you have experienced and how you presently feel about God. But if you truly believe in God, then why does it not show in your life? If you take the necessary steps to break the patterns of feeling the trauma all over again, then there is a huge chance of making a positive change in your life. Do you ever wonder why people have to diet all of the time? Diets work as they should, as a temporary fix. When you start eating again, all the weight, plus more, comes back on your body. That is why we need a healthy lifestyle change rather than a diet.

Give yourself positive affirmations and associate with people who are uplifting. Stop associating with people who have either to validate you or put you down. You can do that by yourself—no help needed, right? If you start feeling good about you, then the opinions of others will no longer matter. You will also find out that a lot of time is wasted on useless opinions because you could have been giving yourself an A+ all along.

...Be relaxed with what you have. Since God assured us, I'll never let you down, never walk off and leave you, we can boldly quote: God is there, ready to help, I'm fearless no matter what. Who or what can get to me?
Hebrews 13:5-6

Chapter 7
Goal Setting

Set realistic goals for yourself. Healthy weight loss occurs at a rate of 1-3 pounds per week on average. Consult a physician or research a healthy rate of weight loss for you. The programs listed in this book for weight loss up to 10 lbs per week are ONLY for jump starting your plan. Do not use the programs more than a week or two at a time. I have presented healthy eating plans for ongoing weight loss and maintenance. I guarantee that if you follow one of the maintenance plans, you will lose weight and keep it off. No need to buy processed foods that can be shipped to your door. Take pride in pampering yourself by cooking. Don't know how to cook? This is a good time to start. There are hundreds of cookbooks waiting for you!

Remember to exercise on a regular basis. A mild plan is 20 minutes per day, 3 times per week. You should really practice doing more than that to remain healthy and physically fit. Drink lots of water. I add lemon juice (a natural diuretic) to my water to help keep my kidneys and liver healthy.

Ready, set, go! Do you have a journal? Yes, you do! I have provided a 30-day journal to get you started. Prayers? Those are included, too! Eating plans? I've got you covered! A food journal? That's part of the package too! Writing down what you eat is a healthy way to keep track of how you are treating yourself.

Give yourself a break and follow one of the plans in this book. The plans are suggestions to get you started. If you have another plan or would like to use something else, then please do. Support groups are available to supplement the transition you are making. Do it for yourself! Love yourself enough to enjoy the beautiful temple God has given you! Trust God, love your neighbor as yourself, and believe all things are possible through God!

We plan the way we want to live, but only GOD makes us able to live it. *Proverbs 16:9*

Chapter 8
Meditation & Journal

Meditation is a very important part of building an everlasting relationship with God. If you trust God with all your heart, mind, and soul, you will give God time to communicate with you each day. We often run through life expecting God to answer our prayers when we do not stop and take time to listen. There are many books and an abundance of information on meditation. If you really want to live free from self, then give yourself a chance with this technique. People have done this for many, many years, and they all say the same thing: "It is worth the time."

Journaling is a faultless process to increase your communication with God and create awareness of yourself. When you write how you are feeling, the rewards are endless. People who take the time to write have a higher success rate than those who say "I do not have time." We have time for whatever we want to do, if we want to do it. *Time belongs to us; we are the ones who choose to use it on things other than taking care of ourselves.* Journal every day and see how great you feel. You will have a written history to mark the progress of your new healthy lifestyle and relationship with God.

I have included 30 days' worth of meditation and journal material for your use. Do not stop there; keep going with it because it really works. I believe in you and know meditation and journaling will help.

Trust God

Romans 12:3

. . . The only accurate way to understand ourselves is by what God is and by what he does for us, not by what we are and what we do for him.

Dear God,

There is no lack or limitation in my life – tomorrow is only a norm right now and is not promised. Today, I must live to be joyful in receiving the Grace and Mercy You have bestowed upon me. God, please show me your will today in all of my goals. Your will be done.

Mark 11:24
Therefore, I tell you, whatever you ask for in prayers believe you have received it, and it will be yours.

Journal – Day 1

Feelings:

_____

_____

_____

Prayer:

_____

_____

_____

Dear God,

I know I am not perfect, and I have to remember that your will may not be what I think it is. The plans you have for my life are revealed to me as you have designed them to be. I know that God wants me to take care of my body, which is my temple. To do this I must live a healthy lifestyle on this earth by eating for nourishment and freeing myself of all ill will towards any of your children.

Mark 12:33
And to love him with all the heart, and with all the understanding, and with all the soul, and with all the strength, and to love his neighbor as himself, is more than all whole burnt offerings and sacrifices.

Journal – Day 2

Feelings:

_____

_____

_____

Prayer:

_____

_____

_____

Dear God,

Make me over again. I know I have had times when you have renewed me without my asking. It has been your Grace and Mercy that brought me through these periods, when I needed you and did not know it. Oh Lord, please restore my faith that I can stand on your will to take care of my temple, the house you gave me to live in, my body. God, please show me peace internally that I may exhibit it externally.

Proverbs 3:5

Trust in the LORD with all thy heart; and lean not unto thy own understanding.

Journal – Day 3

Feelings:

_____

_____

_____

Prayer:

_____

_____

_____

Dear God,

As I continue to pray for God's will to be done in my life, I must discern patterns of my own will. Acknowledging when I am in my own will would lead me to the patience needed to wait on You, God. When I put off until tomorrow what I can do today, it could mean missing an opportunity to do God's will. Knowledge is gained through understanding this. Wisdom is gained through experience. Thy will, not mine, be done.

Proverbs 2:6
For the LORD giveth wisdom: out of his mouth cometh knowledge and understanding.

Journal – Day 4

Feelings:

_____

_____

_____

Prayer:

_____

_____

_____

Dear God,

Exercising alone, even with a healthy eating plan, cannot lead to total physical well-being. I must remember that prayer and meditation are key factors that complete a healthy, wholesome lifestyle. Acknowledging God throughout my day makes everything a success. Thank you, God, for everything, even the things I do not want, such as large hips, love handles, etc. If I thank and acknowledge you for everything, then the path to a healthy lifestyle will be complete.

Proverbs 3:6
In all thy ways acknowledge him, and he shall make your paths straight.

Journal – Day 5

Feelings:

_____

_____

_____

Prayer:

_____

_____

_____

Dear God,

I am praying that I can love myself enough to gain perfect health. Through your Grace and Mercy, I know that all things are possible. I cannot waver nor can I put off until tomorrow what I can do today. Your Grace is sufficient for any challenge that is before me. I must remember to love myself as I love you, God, as I am made in your likeness.

I Corinthians 13:10
But when that which is perfect is come, then that which is in part shall be done away.

Journal – Day 6

Feelings:

_____

_____

_____

Prayer:

_____

_____

_____

Day 7

Dear God,

Unmanageability is a trait that has to be surrendered to God many times during the day. We have to seek God's will in all things and have the courage to act on it. What is more important is having the tenacity to be courageous and meet the goal of having a healthy body. We are not alone in this, God is *always* here. Be strong in faith; let God remove unmanageable behavior.

Romans 1:12
That is, that you and I may be mutually encouraged by each other's faith.

Journal – Day 7

Feelings:

_____

_____

_____

Prayer:

_____

_____

_____

Dear God,

Reliance upon self does not work, even if I keep trying to convince myself that it does. God, please reveal your will to me so that I may understand that it is the only way. Worrying about the day's activities takes me to places where I really do not want to go. I must remember that in all of the times I have tried to control my life, worrying has been a part of it. Lord God, you do not give us any more then we can handle. You do not bring the extra bags—we do.

Matthew 6:27
Who of you by worrying can add a single hour to their life?

Journal – Day 8

Feelings:

_____

_____

_____

Prayer:

_____

_____

_____

Dear God,

I cannot do anything without you. I keep trying to plan my day without asking for your will. I know your will is not for me to continue to harm myself. It is for me to love myself more than anything or anyone except You, God. How I view the world is a direct reflection of how I see myself. The beauty within is revealed only when I want to see it. However it is your will for me always to see it, because I am made in your likeness.

Matthew 6:22
The light of the body is the eye: if therefore thine eye be single, thy whole body shall be full of light.

Journal - Day 9

Feelings:

_____

_____

_____

Prayer:

_____

_____

_____

Dear God,

The more I want to stop eating, the more I eat. I pray that I can focus on your will and not on what I am eating. I pray that you continue to enlighten me with your words, Lord, and that I live by those words and focus on them more than I focus on food. Jesus fasted 40 days and 40 nights.

Matthew 4:4
But he answered and said, It is written, Man shall not live by bread alone, but by every word that comes from the mouth of God.

Journal – Day 10

Feelings:

_____

_____

_____

Prayer:

_____

_____

_____

Dear God,

If only I could...if only you could...I've been
trying...I can't seem to . . . ., etc. These are all
familiar sayings that we use to bargain with God.
How long have you been trying to reach that goal
of losing weight? The operative word is "you." The
fact is that we ask for God's will, but turn to
ourselves. How many more goals are you going to
set? Let go and believe God has set the goals—
you just have to know this is true.

Matthew 4:7
Do not put the Lord your God to the test.

Journal – Day 11

Feelings:

_____

_____

_____

Prayer:

_____

_____

_____

Dear God,

Today, I know that your spirit guides me. It is
only when I think I know more than you, God, that
I go back to my unproductive way of thinking.
Well, maybe it is not unproductive, because this
way of thinking helps me get back to you, God.
The Spirit of God guides me always. I love God
more than anything I need or want. I only need to
know God's Spirit; all else will come naturally.

I Corinthians 2:12
We have not received the spirit of the world but
the Spirit who is from God, that we may
understand what God has freely given us.

Journal – Day 12

Feelings:

_____

_____

_____

Prayer:

_____

_____

_____

Dear God,

My lack of discipline is a sign of my desire to control my life when I focus on changing me rather than on pleasing you, God. I will take care of my temple and stop using it as a repository for my past, my pain, and my fears. My Temple (body) should be a reflection of the love I have for you and an example of the love you have for me.

Isaiah 65:16
Whoever invokes a blessing in the land will do so by the God of truth; he who takes an oath in the land will swear by the God of truth. For the past troubles will be forgotten and hidden from my eyes.

Journal – Day 13

Feelings:

_____

_____

_____

Prayer:

_____

_____

_____

Dear God,

Learning to remember that you are the source of
my supply is a very sufficient act on my behalf,
when I do it. The problem is I forget that God is
the source of my supply; therefore, I fall short
of knowing my needs have been met. God, thy will
is done always, even when I take the long way
around and put my selfish motives in front of
what you want me to do. I must humbly succumb
to your will, because that is really all there is,
according to your Word.

Psalm 149:4
For the LORD taketh pleasure in his people: he
will beautify the meek with salvation.

Journal – Day 14

Feelings:

_____

_____

_____

Prayer:

_____

_____

_____

Dear God,

Whispers from my soul tell me that all I need is God, yet I am unresolved as to why I am leaning towards anything but God. I love You, God, and it has been a journey to find out that the handling of my life has always belonged to God. The pen I use to write to you represents my heart. God, please let what is in my heart show in my means of keeping my temple, healthy and whole. God is deep in my heart. I have faith that I will know this as each day begins.

Proverbs 3:3
Let not mercy and truth forsake thee: bind them about thy neck; write them upon the table of thine heart:

Journal – Day 15

Feelings:

_____

_____

_____

Prayer:

_____

_____

Dear God,

Tomorrow will take care of itself. Today is the
day God has made, and my needs are met. Whew!
Thank God this is sufficient information for me
to make it through the day. There is peace in
knowing that God is the source of my supply and
that everything comes through God. The question
is will I follow this way? My temple (body) is
God's House for my soul. I must follow His way to
take care of it.

I Corinthians 14:20
Brethren, be not children in understanding:
howbeit in malice be ye children, but in
understanding be men.

Journal – Day 16

Feelings:

_____

_____

_____

Prayer:

_____

_____

_____

Dear God,

Obedience is the key in my life today. Loving my temple (body) is enough because you love me much more. God, seeking your will is not always the simplest thing to do, only because you give me free will. God, please show me how peaceful it is to be obedient to you. Your will for me is sufficient, and the guidance you give me is enough for every moment of the day

Matthew 5:12
Rejoice, and be glad, for great is your reward in heaven.

Journal – Day 17

Feelings:

_____

_____

_____

Prayer:

_____

_____

_____

Dear God,

Why don't I know that your Grace and Mercy are sufficient? Or, maybe I know this, but am not living like I know it. God, your will for me is greater than anything I can imagine. My temple is designed by you and given to me as a precious gift. God, please show me how to take care of this precious gift and to love you enough to do your will. Let me show you how much Your Mercy and Grace mean to me.

Philippians 4:6
Do not be anxious about anything, but in everything by prayer and petition, with thanksgiving, present your requests to God.

Journal – Day 18
Feelings:

_____

_____

_____

Prayer:

_____

_____

_____

Dear God,

My life is designed by God. However, I continue
to live as though outside influences can make me
feel any different. The pain I think I am escaping
from through food is only an illusion. I never feel
better, just different, and the pain does not go
away after I eat food. My inner being is still
hurting. Lord, please continue to do your healing.
Help me take care of my body.

Ephesians 4:4-6
There is one body, and one Spirit, even as ye are
called in one hope of your calling; One Lord, one
faith, one baptism, One God and Father of all,
who is above all, and through all, and in you all.

Journal – Day 19

Feelings:

_____

_____

_____

Prayer:

_____

_____

_____

Dear God,

Your grace is the power you have exalted upon me. Lord, there are days when I turn to food, when I know I should turn to you. Your Grace and Mercy are sufficient for my needs. God, I need to know how to practice this in my life. Your power is the way for me. Let me be an example of your will. Thy will, not mine, be done.

Ephesians 1:19
. . . and his incomparably great power for us who believe. That power is like the working of his mighty strength.

Journal – Day 20

Feelings:

_____

_____

_____

Prayer:

_____

_____

_____

Dear God,

Doing the right thing is simple, but not always
easy. Being righteous is being controlled by Faith
in God's word. The righteous live in Faith. Faith is
the belief in things unseen. We know God is here.
Turn to Him instead of outside influences, such as
unhealthy eating habits. Be mindful of the Power
of God. Seek righteousness by doing the right
thing in his Word.

Romans 1:17
For therein is the righteousness of God revealed
from faith to faith: as it is written, the just shall
live by faith.

Journal - Day 21

Feelings:

_____

_____

_____

Prayer:

_____

_____

_____

Dear God,

Stress makes me feel lonely and reactionary. I
must turn to you in my time of need. Your will is
the only "Food" I need. Your Grace and Mercy
have blessed me this far. There is no reason for
me to think that I will be without you now. I know
you are always with me. I just have to call upon
you instead of these outside influences, such as
food. Restore me, God, so that I can always call
on you.

Psalm 31:19
How great is your goodness, which you have
stored up for those who fear you, which you
bestow in the sight of men . . .

Journal – Day 22

Feelings:

_____

_____

_____

Prayer:

_____

_____

_____

Day 23

Dear God,

The lessons in life always lead me back to God.
The food I eat, the clothes I wear, the means to
live on this earth are all blessings from God. I
must remember these things are graciously given
to me through God's grace and mercy. As we all
have heard, I don't have to worry "'bout a thing."

Matthew 6:25
Therefore I say unto you, Take no thought for
your life, what ye shall eat, or what ye shall drink;
nor yet for your body, what you shall put on. Is
not the life more than meat, and the body than
raiment?

Journal – Day 23

Feelings:

_____

_____

_____

Prayer:

_____

_____

_____

Dear God,

Please let me know that I am enough. God, I pray
that I can learn to love myself, my inner being,
enough to love my outside too. When I eat for
comfort, I block You out; when I think I can eat
to satisfy a need, I block you out; when I eat for
any compulsive reason, I block You out. I pray
that I can remember that you supply my needs, all
of them, including food. I do not need to use food
as a means to disguise you because you are what I
need.

Matthew 6:8
Be not ye therefore like unto them: for your
Father knoweth what things ye have need of,
before ye ask him.

Journal – Day 24

Feelings:

_____

_____

_____

Prayer:

_____

_____

_____

Dear God,

Thank you for the laughter; the ability to laugh at myself is possible only through Your Grace and Mercy. I have dieted a lot and to no avail; I gain the weight back and then some. I must love the pain within, laugh in the face of adversity, and know that God has me in his plan. God bless my soul and show me how to love me in spite of myself. Laugh, Love, Live.

Matthew 5:44
But I say unto you, Love your enemies, bless them that curse you, do good to them that hate you, and pray for them which despitefully use you, and persecute you.

Journal – Day 25

Feelings:

_____

_____

_____

Prayer:

_____

_____

_____

Day 25

Dear God,

I take my life for granted and live each day as though I know better than you what is promised the next day. Today is all I know about. I know that I have never been able to see tomorrow, but my ego tells me that it is coming. I must do all things today that please you, including taking care of my temple, because only you know about tomorrow.

Matthew 6:34
Take therefore no thought for the morrow: for the morrow shall take thought for the things of itself.

Journal – Day 26

Feelings:

_____

_____

_____

Prayer:

_____

_____

_____

Dear God,

There is peace in knowing there is a power greater than myself that I can trust. I must remember that believing in this knowledge of God's power should not be an option. My heart must have the desire to do the right thing to take care of my temple. You are my rock, and there is no easier softer way than you. I will trust in you without reservation.

Isaiah 26:4
Trust in the Lord forever, for the Lord is the Rock eternal.

Journal – Day 27

Feelings:

_____

_____

_____

Prayer:

_____

_____

_____

Dear God,

Please forgive me for doubting you. I sometimes forget that you are all powerful, all knowing, all places at all times. When I turn to food for comfort, I block your blessings for me. The plan you have designed for me is unknown, and I must do my best to stay on track with it as life goes by. Taking this path helps me discern your will for me.

Romans 15:5
May the God who gives you endurance and encouragement give you a spirit of unity among yourselves as you follow Christ.

Journal – Day 28

Feelings:

_____

_____

_____

Prayer:

_____

_____

Dear God,

Love is the greatest gift. Love does not doubt, love is full of faith, love trusts, love conquers, love hopes. God is all of these things. Why do I turn to anything other than God whose Grace and Mercy are sufficient? What could possibly give me more pleasure? We may think other things can grant us what *may* be equivalent, but that is so far from the truth. God is Love, and that is all there is.

I Corinthians 13:7
Love bears all things, believes all things, hopes all things, and endures all things.

Journal – Day 29

Feelings:

_____

_____

_____

Prayer:

_____

_____

_____

Dear God,

Lovely, admirable, pure, noble are all the things I must believe about myself. After all, God believes that about me. I must continue to praise Him and to show love towards myself and others. Peace comes from within. Bring forth the Joy into the inner place as you show love outwardly.

Ephesians 4:8-10
Wherefore he said, when he ascended up on high, he led captivity captive, and gave gifts unto men. (Now that he ascended, what is it but that he also descended first into the lower parts of the earth? He that descended is the same also that ascended far above all heavens, that he might fill all things.)

Journal – Day 30

Feelings:

_____

_____

_____

Prayer:

_____

_____

_____

Go to God for Discipline

Chapter 9
Meal & Exercise Plans

I have dieted for most of my life. You would probably say that I am a professional dieter. I find one that works for me and forget where I put it; or I may get tired of the same old plan and want to try something new that works, too! Well, I know many people like me who want to have that successful plan at their fingertips. You Got It! I have compiled many of the plans that have come across my kitchen table. We hope you find this to be helpful and that you will share it with your friends.

All plans are only examples of foods to eat. Of course, comparable foods will provide the same results. Each plan consists of three to four choices for breakfast, lunch, and dinner. Remember, you are gearing towards a permanent fix, not a temporary one. Dieting is a waste of time; God has other things for you to do. When you are done with this, pass it on so someone else can get help too!

If your metabolism is slow, then you would choose a plan that has fewer carbohydrates in the grain and starch families. Be sure to get your BMI (Body Metabolic Index) by using the hyperlinks below, in order to choose the plan that will achieve the greatest results. Please remember that results vary based on body type. Weigh yourself once a week and join a support group! CONSULT YOUR PHYSICIAN BEFORE STARTING ANY EATING PLAN!

Some of us diet for special occasions, as part of our life routine, or because of health reasons. On the following pages you will find an eating plan that fits your lifestyle, giving you the results desired. This should be a lifestyle change for continuous health. After you have reached your goal weight, look at the maintenance plan so that you will not have to go through this again! If you call on *God* and adopt a good food plan that is right for you, success is guaranteed forever, and you should never have to diet again.

Honor God, Eat Well, and Enjoy a Healthy Life!

(Note: substitute any meat w/ a serving of tofu or 3 egg whites
Vegans: substitute all dairy and meats w/ tofu, soy yogurt, and soy milk)

Measuring Definition:

Tbs or Tbsp - Tablespoon
Tsp - Teaspoon
2 oz - 1/8 cup
4 oz - ¼ cup
8 oz - 1 cup

BMI

To get your BMI, access the websites listed below.

Adults: http://www.changeone.com/gen-con/bmicalculator.jhtml;sessionid=DHLETYD41D SJQCTENILSGYIKMRVBOIZF

Youth: http://www.kidshealth.org/teen/food_fitness/wellbeing/weight_height.html

The following eating plans should be used to jumpstart a new regimen for eating healthily. The exercise plans can be used indefinitely. There are numerous exercise plans, food menus, trainers, nutritionists, gyms, and other means to keep you active and healthy. The goal is to put God first, no matter what you do. Enjoy! Your success is guaranteed if you trust and rely upon God through the process and forever.

Easy Lo-Cal Eating * 1,200 Calories per Day *
Lose up to 7 lbs each week

Breakfast
(Choose One Daily)

2 Egg Whites, 1 Yolk ½ Banana	½ Orange ½ Cup Chicken	1 Cup Plain Yogurt ½ Banana, 3 Pineapple Slices, 1 tsp Coconut Extract

Lunch
(Choose One Daily)

¾ Cup Pasta 2 oz Chicken 5 Tbs. Italian Dressing	½ Bag Cooked Ramen Noodles ½ Cup Each Cooked Snow Peas & Broccoli	4 oz Diced Turkey 1 tsp. Light Vinaigrette 1 Orange

Dinner
(Choose One Daily)

4 Oz Chicken Breast ½ Each Grapes, Berries, and Pineapple ½ Cup Celery 1 Tbs Dressing	4 Oz Chicken Breast ½ Cup Broccoli 3 Asparagus Spears 2 Oz Cheese ½ Cup Grapes	8 oz Group Turkey 2 Tbs Seasoning 1 Cup Each Spinach and Celery 3 Sliced Mushrooms 2 Tsp Lite Vinaigrette

Snack
(Eat anytime desired)
1 cup plain yogurt or 1 serving of fruit (apple, orange, banana, 8oz strawberries, 3 pineapple slices) or 1 cup of spinach

Exercise Program:

30 Minutes Daily Cardio (Choose One: Walking, Cycling, Aerobics Class/Tape)
15 Minutes 4 times per week Toning (Resistance Band, Circuit Training, Free Weights)

Low Carb * 60 Carbs Low/140 High Per Day *
Lose up to 6 lbs each week
Alternate Low and High Carbs Each Day (Ex:
Mon – Low Carb, Tue – High Carb, Etc.)

Breakfast
(Choose One Daily)

4 Egg Whites, 1 tsp oil, 2 oz cheese, 8 oz strawberries Low Carb	10 Oz Fat Free Plain Yogurt, 1 Medium Apple, 3 Tbs Chopped Nuts Low Carb	1 Cup Fresh Fruit or 4 Oz Fruit Juice 1 Cup Whole Grain Cereal, $\frac{3}{4}$ Cup Fat-Free Milk High Carb	2 Whole Wheat Waffles, 1 $\frac{1}{2}$ Tbs Maple Syrup 1 Cup Fruit High Carb

Lunch
(Choose One Daily)

1 Low Carb Protein Bar or Shake 2 Cups Raw	6 Oz Tuna or Bun less Burger	3 Tbs Peanut Butter 1 Tbs All	2 Oz Chicken or Tuna 3 Cups

Veggies 2 Tbs Low Carb Dip 1 boiled Egg 1 Tbs Mayonnaise *Low Carb*	3 Cups Mixed Veggie Salad 3 Tbs Low Carb Dressing *Low Carb*	Fruit Preserves 2 Slices Whole Wheat Bread 6 Baby Carrots *High Carb*	Mixed Salad 2 Tbs Dressing 1 Medium Baked or Sweet Potato 1 Tbs Sour Cream *High Carb*

Dinner
(Choose One Daily)

4 Oz Steak, 1Tsp Spice Rub; 12 Asparagus, lemon 1 Oz Blue Cheese *Low Carb*	4 Oz Chicken Breast $\frac{1}{2}$ Cup Broccoli 3 Asparagus Spears 2 Oz Cheese $\frac{1}{2}$ Cup Grapes *Low Carb*	1 Cup Low Fat Chili w/out Beans 2 Tbs Sour Cream 1 Ear Corn 2 Cups Bell Pepper	$\frac{3}{4}$ Cup Whole Wheat Pasta $\frac{1}{4}$ Cup Pasta Sauce 1 Tbs Parmesan 2 Cups Mixed Salad; 2 Tbs

		High Carb	Dressing; 4 Oz Sliced Deli Meat High Carb

Snack - None

Exercise Program: 30 Minutes Daily (Choose One: Walking, Cycling, Aerobics Class/Tape, Yoga, Pilates)

*1300 Calorie menu * Lose up to 8 lbs each week

Breakfast
(Choose One Daily)

1 frozen breakfast sandwich (up to 300 calories) , 1 cup/piece of fruit	1 protein bar or shake (up to 200 calories) 1 piece/cup of fruit	1 packet of Oatmeal or $\frac{3}{4}$ cup cold cereal (up to 180 calories) 1 piece/cup fruit $\frac{1}{2}$ cup fat free or non fat milk

Lunch
(Choose One Daily)

4 oz turkey, 2 slices light bread, 2 tsp light mayo, lettuce and tomato 1oz pretzels 1 cup baby carrots	6 Oz Shrimp 1/3 cup cocktail sauce 2 cups mixed salad, 2 tsp light dressing 2 short breadsticks	1 cup turkey chili 1 oz baked chips 1 cup bell pepper 2tbs light dressing

Dinner
(Choose One Daily)

4 Oz roasted chicken breast, 1tbs cranberry sauce 1 small sweet potato 1 cup broccoli	4 oz shrimp or salmon 1tbs teriyaki sauce ½ cup brown rice 1 cup snow peas or Asian vegetables	4 Oz lean beef or lamb chop 1 tsp spice rub ½ cup whole grain rice 1 cup grilled or steamed vegetables

Snack – Choose two daily: 2 reduced fat cheese sticks or ½ cup fat free yogurt w/berries; 1 cup flavored light yogurt or 3 chocolate wafer cookies w/ 1 cup fat free milk; 2tbs each nuts and dried fruit or 1 piece of fruit or 1tbs peanut butter. *NOTE: You can substitute the lunch or dinner w/a low-fat frozen meal that has 300 calories or less along w/2 cups tossed salad and 2tbs dressing.*

Exercise Program: 30 Minutes Daily (Choose One: Walking, Cycling, Aerobics Class/Tape, Yoga, Pilates)

Exotic Meal Plan - Lose up to 5lbs per week

Breakfast
(Choose One Daily)

2 slices raisin bread ½ tbsp low fat cream cheese Coffee or Tea	¾ cup bran flake cereal; 8 oz nonfat milk; 1 small banana Coffee or Tea	1 egg and two egg whites or 4 egg whites; ½ onions, tomatoes and peppers (combined), 1tbsp olive oil 1 cup melon cubes 8oz nonfat milk	1 whole wheat low fat English muffin; 1tbsp fat free margarine; 1 cup melon cubes Coffee or Tea

Lunch
(Choose One Daily)

2 medium soft tacos w/ground beef; shredded lettuce, cheese and taco sauce 1 cup	2oz roast beef; 2 slices of light rye or wheat bread; mustard, tomato, pickle 1 cup salad	1 veggie burger, 1 whole wheat pita bread; 1 slice reduced fat cheese; onion/tomato/mustard 1 cup salad greens w/1tbsp fat free salad dressing 1 pear	3oz tuna; 1tbsp light mayo; chopped onion to taste – mix salad; 1 slice fat

salad greens w/1tbsp fat free salad dressing	greens w/1tbsp fat free salad dressing 1 apple		free or reduced fat cheese; 2 slices whole wheat bread; 1 cup salad greens w/1tbsp fat free salad dressing 1 pear

Dinner
(Choose One Daily)

1 6oz baked chicken breast; 1 cup steamed green vegetables; 2 cups salad greens w/1tbsp fat free salad	4oz baked fish; 1 cup 1 cup steamed green vegetables; 2 cups salad greens w/1tbsp fat free salad dressing	4oz turkey breast; $\frac{1}{2}$ baked potato or sweet potato; 1 cup steamed green vegetables; 1 cup salad greens w/1tbsp fat free	4oz pork chop (baked or pan fried w/nonfat cooking spray); 1 cup steamed green vegetables; 2 cups salad greens

dressing		salad dressing	w/1tbsp fat free salad dressing

Snack – select two daily: plain nonfat yogurt, 1 cup raw vegetables, 1tbsp walnuts or almonds

30 Minutes Daily (Choose One: Walking, Cycling, Aerobics Class/Tape)
15 Minutes toning 4 times per week (Resistance Band, Circuit Training, Free Weights)

1,200 calories per day, lose up to *12 lbs in three weeks*

Breakfast
(Choose One Daily)

4 egg whites scrambled 1 $\frac{1}{2}$ cup vegetables 1 tangerine	1 cup low fat cottage cheese w/veggies $\frac{1}{2}$ pear	6 oz plain nonfat yogurt; 1 tbsp high fiber cereal; $\frac{1}{2}$ cup berries

Lunch
(Choose One Daily)

4oz turkey burger; 1 slice reduced fat cheese; mustard; 4 cups salad; 2 tbsp low fat or fat free dressing	8oz chicken $\frac{1}{4}$ cup chopped celery; 1 tbsp chopped walnuts or almonds; 1tbsp light mayo; 4 cups salad	2 oz roast beef; 1 slice ; 1 slice reduced fat cheese; 2 cups salad; 2 tbsp low fat or fat free dressing

Dinner
(Choose One Daily)

3 oz salmon; 3 cups green vegetables	3 oz lamb chops; 1 tomato; 3 cups lettuce; oil and vinegar to taste	3oz sirloin steak; 1/3 cup each mushroom, onions, bell pepper sautéed in olive oil; 2 cups steamed green vegetables

Snack – 1 cup of sugar free gelatin, 2 tbsp low fat whipped cream & ½ cup of blueberries or raspberries; or 1 cup fat free milk & 1tbsp cocoa mix w/ice in a blender.

Exercise Program: 30 Minutes Daily (Choose One: Walking, Cycling, Aerobics Class/Tape, Yoga, Pilates)

Balanced Meal Plan lose up to 1 lb per day

Breakfast
(Choose One Daily)

1 whole grain low fat English muffin; 2tbsp peanut butter; 1 tsp fruit spread; ½ cup fat free milk 1 small banana	¼ cup cooked steel cut oatmeal; ½ tbsp dried fruit; 1 tbsp almonds	½ cup high fiber cereal; ¾ cup blueberries; ¾ cup fat free milk

Lunch
(Choose One Daily)

3 oz turkey; 3 cups green salad; 1 cup baby carrots; 1 slice low fat cheese; 1 tbsp fat free ranch dressing; 1 whole wheat roll; 1 orange	2 oz grilled chicken; 2 slices light whole wheat bread; 1 oz low-fat cheese; 1 cup baby carrots; 2 tsp balsamic vinaigrette; 1 medium apple	3 oz roast beef; 1 oz low fat cheese; lettuce, 1tsp light mayo; ½ pita ½ cup veggies; 1 cup melon

Dinner
(Choose One Daily)

5 oz salmon; ½ cup brown rice; 10 asparagus spears; 1 orange	3 oz roasted chicken; 2 cups green vegetables; 1 baked potato or sweet potato	6 oz grilled red snapper or pork tenderloin; 1 cup green vegetables; ½ tbsp olive oil; 1 cup pineapple

Snack – Choose one daily - 2 graham crackers w/2tbsp peanut butter; 6 whole grain crackers w/ 1oz low fat cheese; ½ cup low fat pudding; ½ whole grain bagel, 1 tbsp low fat cream cheese; 6 oz low fat yogurt; ½ cup blueberries w/8 almonds; toaster size-small waffle w/ ¼ cup low fat cottage cheese 1 tsp fruit spread Exercise Program: 30 Minutes Daily (Choose One: Walking, Cycling, Aerobics Class/Tape, Yoga, Pilates)

Lose up to 10lbs per week

Breakfast
(Choose One Daily)

2 eggs, fresh basil; 1 tsp parmesan ; 1 sliced tomato; 1 slice whole-grain bread	1 cup fortified whole-grain cereal with nuts; ½ cup fat free milk; 1 orange	½ cup high protein whole grain cereal; 1 cup fat free milk; ½ cup berries

Lunch
(Choose One Daily)

3 oz tuna or salmon; 2 tsp light mayo; 2 slices light whole grain bread; 1 cup tomato soup; ½ cup bell pepper	3 oz grilled fish; 2 cups salad, 3 tbsp light dressing; 1 small whole-grain roll; 1tsp butter	3 oz grilled chicken; 2 cups salad, 3 tbsp light dressing; 1 small whole-grain roll; 1tsp butter

Dinner
(Choose One Daily)

3 oz chicken, 2 tsp peanut oil; 2 cups Asian mixed vegetables; 1 tbsp teriyaki sauce; 1 cup brown rice; 2 tbsp sliced almonds	1 ½ cups pasta, 2 cups roasted vegetables, 2 tsp olive oil, ¼ cup parmesan or low fat feta cheese	4" French bread, ½ cup tomato sauce, 3 oz mozzarella; 3 cups salad; 1 tsp olive oil, vinegar

Snack – Choose two daily – 1 oz almonds & ½ cup vegetable slices; 1 cup/piece fruit & ½ cup low fat cottage cheese; 1 stick string cheese, ½ cup vegetable slices & 3 whole grain crackers

Exercise Program: 30 to 60 Minutes Daily - Power Walking, include hills; Break walks into 10 minute intervals if necessary

Lose up to 7 lbs per week

Breakfast
(Choose One Daily)

2 eggs, 1 egg white; 1 tsp canola margarine; 1 cup berries	2 large whole-grain pancakes , 1 tsp canola margarine; 12/ cup sugar free yogurt; ½ cup berries	½ cup high protein whole grain cereal; 1 cup fat free milk; ½ cup berries

Lunch
(Choose One Daily)

4 oz sliced turkey; 1 whole wheat tortilla; ¼ avocado; lettuce, diced tomatoes, salsa and cilantro	4oz chicken; 2 cups cabbage; ¼ cup orange slices; 2 tbsp almonds and rice vinegar; 1 tbsp sesame seeds and sesame oil; green onion	5 oz cooked salmon over 3 cups baby spinach; 3 artichoke hearts; 5 olives; 1 tbsp nuts; 1 tbsp vinaigrette and dill

Dinner
(Choose One Daily)

5oz grilled pork tenderloin; 1 baked sweet potato, 2-3 cups tossed salad, 1tbsp light vinaigrette	4 oz halibut w/ 1/3 cup mango salsa; 2 cups baby spinach; 2 red onions; 1tbsp feta cheese; 1 tbsp white wine vinegar	5 oz grilled flank steak; 3 cups fresh broccoli w/1tsp pine nuts; ½ tbsp olive oil and lemon juice; 2 cups tossed salad w/1 tbsp light vinaigrette

Snack – Choose two daily - ½ cup sugar free fruit yogurt; 4 dried apricot halves & 4walnut halves; 1 green apple sliced; 2 tbsp chopped fruit; 1 celery stalk & 2 tbsp peanut butter; ½ cup sugar free yogurt & ½ cup berries; ½ cup baby carrots & 2 tbsp hummus

Exercise Program – Choose one daily - 30 to 60 Minutes Daily - Power Walking, include hills; Break walks into 10 minute intervals if necessary; Cycling, Aerobics Class/Tape, Yoga, Pilates

Lose up to 7 lbs per week

Breakfast
(Choose One Daily)

1 hard boiled egg 1 small bran muffin 1 serving fruit	1 cup low fat cottage cheese 1tsp sliced almonds 1 serving fruit	1 whole wheat English muffin; 1 slice Canadian bacon; 1 slice low fat cheese; 1 serving fruit

Lunch
(Choose One Daily)

8 oz baked white fish ½ cup boiled red potatoes 2 tbsp vinegar 1 tbsp olive oil 1 cup green	1 can tuna drained; 3 tbsp rice vinegar 1tsp soy sauce; 1 diced cucumber; 8 whole wheat crackers	1 bar-b-que *sandwich (*6 oz ground beef or turkey, ½ cup apple cider vinegar; 2 tbsp ketchup, 1 tbsp Worcestershire sauce, salt & pepper; 2 tbsp Dijon mustard, 1 whole wheat bun) 1 ½ cups mixed vegetables

Dinner
(Choose One Daily)

1 slice cheese pizza; 3 cups salad w/2 tbsp vinegar; 1 tbsp oil	6 oz turkey breast or fish 12 oz winter squash, heated w/3tbsp balsamic vinegar; 2 tsp extra-virgin olive oil; salt and pepper; 1 ½ cups broccoli	8 oz cooked chicken breast w/cider vinegar sauce* 1 ½ cups spinach (*2 tsp olive oil, ½ chopped onion, 3 tbsp apple cider vinegar; 1 cup canned low-salt chicken broth – sauté onion in oil, add vinegar and broth, stir.

Snack – Choose two daily - 1 cup veggies, 3 tbsp light ranch dressing; 1 stick string cheese; 3 whole grain crackers, 2 tbsp light cream cheese; 1 cup broth based soup; ½ cup All-Bran cereal, ½ cup fat free milk; ½ small apple w/tbsp peanut butter

Exercise Program – Choose one daily - 30 to 60 Minutes Daily - Power Walking, include hills; Break walks into 10 minute intervals if necessary; Cycling, Aerobics Class/Tape, Yoga, Pilates

Lose up to 14 lbs in 10 days

Breakfast
(Choose One Daily)

2 eggs w/ 2 tsp olive oil 1 slice avocado, salsa; 1 whole wheat tortilla	½ cup whole grain cereal 1 cup fat free milk	2 poached eggs 1 cup mushrooms sautéed in 2tsp olive oil

Lunch
(Choose One Daily)

3 oz rotisserie chicken breast; 2 cups greens, ½ cup white beans, ½ cup artichoke hearts, 1 tbsp each pine nuts and olive oil vinaigrette	¼ cup each green beans, diced tomato, chickpeas, fresh parsley, 2 tbsp olives, 2 tbsp vinaigrette	3 oz salmon 2 cups salad, 1 tbsp olives, 1 tbsp olive-oil vinaigrette 1 whole wheat pita

Dinner
(Choose One Daily)

4 oz grilled or broiled flank steak prepared with 1tbsp olive oil ½ cup wiled rice; 1 tbsp diced roasted red pepper and goat cheese; 1 ½ cup broccoli	4oz grilled or broiled tuna steak w/lemon ½ cup whole wheat pasta 1 ½ cups asparagus, 1 tsp lemon, 1 tsp olive oil	4 oz chicken breast marinated w/ 2tsp olive oil vinaigrette 1 ½ cups roasted vegetables

Snack – Choose two daily - 10 almonds; 1 laughing cow mini baby cell cheese; 1 cup sliced red bell peppers; 2 tbsp peanut butter w/celery; 3 tbsp hummus w/bell peppers, broccoli & tomato

Exercise Program – Choose one daily - 30 to 60 Minutes Daily - Power Walking, include hills; Break walks into 10 minute intervals if necessary; Cycling, Aerobics Class/Tape, Yoga, Pilates;

Lose up to 3 lbs in 7 days

Breakfast
(Choose One Daily)

3 ½ tbsp protein powder 1 cup fat free milk ¼ cup fruit juice 1 cup fruit ½ banana 1//4 tsp cinnamon or nutmeg; blend	3 egg whites prepared w/nonfat cooking spray 2 slices turkey bacon	1 cup low fat cottage cheese 2 tsp chopped nuts ½ cup berries

Lunch
(Choose One Daily)

2 tbsp peanut butter w/ 1 tbsp fruit spread 2 slices light wheat bread 1 cup celery sticks	1 ½ cups cooked whole grain pasta Marinara sauce; 1 tbsp parmesan cheese 2 cups mixed greens; 2 slices red onion; 2 tbsp fat-free dressing	2 cups low-fat lentil soup 4 cups mixed greens; ¼ cup croutons, 2 tbsp parmesan cheese, 3 tbsp fat-free dressing

Dinner
(Choose One Daily)

4 oz grilled or broiled flank steak prepared with 1tbsp olive oil $\frac{1}{2}$ cup wiled rice; 1 tbsp diced roasted red pepper and goat cheese; 1 $\frac{1}{2}$ cup broccoli	3 oz roasted chicken; 2 cups green vegetables; 1 baked potato or sweet potato	4 oz chicken breast marinated w/ 2tsp olive oil vinaigrette 1 $\frac{1}{2}$ cups roasted vegetables

Snack – Choose one daily - 1 apple; 10 baked tortilla chips w/ $\frac{1}{4}$ cup salsa; 1 cup low-fat vegetable soup; 2 tbsp almonds; 3 slices turkey breast; 1 deviled egg prepared with 1 tbsp fat-free may

Exercise Program – Choose one daily - 30 to 60 Minutes Daily - Power Walking, include hills; Break walks into 10 minute intervals if necessary; Cycling, Aerobics Class/Tape, Yoga, Pilates; routines can be split between the morning and evening, i.e., 30 minutes in morning and 30 minutes in evening

Maintenance

With a lot of other eating plans, the fix is temporary, and once you start eating "normal" foods again, then you will gain the weight back. Also, I wonder why we care so little about ourselves that we buy pre-packaged food and have someone deliver it to us so that we can lose weight. How long do you think that will last? As soon as you stop eating that food, oops, it is highly possible that the weight will come back!

Remember that you will do a lot of work to get the weight off and to get emotionally and mentally healthy too! You are strengthening your relationship with God, and you must continue to rely on him. Commitment is the key to maintenance in life. If you commit to your daily practice of prayer, meditation, and journaling, then the chances of your having to start over again are slim to none.

Remember that God is here for you! Choose what works in your life and live it to the fullest! Healthy living is a choice. Choose to be healthy in mind, body, and spirit.

Breakfast

(Choose One Daily)

1 ½ cups whole grain cereal 1 cup low fat milk 1 banana	2 poached eggs 1 slice whole wheat toast 1tsp jelly	1 ½ cups cooked oatmeal 1 cup low-fat milk 1 cup berries	2 each 4" pancakes 2 tbsp maple syrup 2 slices Canadian bacon 1 cup berries

Lunch

(Choose One Daily)

3 oz grilled chicken breast 3 cups mixed greens 2 tbsp grated fat free grated cheese 2 tbsp low fat dressing 1 tangerine 1 cup low fat milk 1 miniature candy bar	2 slices whole grain bread 3 oz lean turkey breast 2 cups salad greens 1 tbsp light dressing 1 cup berries	3 oz water packed tuna 2 tbsp light mayo 1 tbsp chopped onion 2 slices light whole wheat bread 1 oz mozzarella cheese 1 peach	1 cup tomato soup with ½ cup diced tomatoes 2 slices whole wheat bread 1 oz low fat sharp cheddar cheese ½ cup cottage cheese

Dinner
(Choose One Daily)

3 oz salmon steak 2 cups spinach 1 tbsp light dressing 1 small baked potato 1 tbsp light sour cream ½ cup light ice cream	1 cup angel hair pasta, ½ cup tomato sauce 1 slice whole wheat toast, 1 tsp olive oil w/fresh garlic 2 cups romaine lettuce 1tbsp light dressing 1 chocolate covered graham cracker	2 whole wheat flour tortillas 2 oz grilled chicken breast 1 cup chopped lettuce ¼ cup each low fat sharp cheddar cheese ¼ cup salsa 2 tbsp sour cream	3 oz beef tenderloin and 2 cups of vegetables 2 tbsp teriyaki sauce 1/3 cup steamed brown rice 1 cup cubed melon 3 vanilla wafers

Snack – select one daily: 10 almonds, 1 oz string cheese, 10 grapes; 1 hard boiled egg, 1 oz lean ham, 1 orange; ½ whole wheat bagel, 1 tbsp light cream cheese, 4 oz vegetable juice; ¼ cup low fat yogurt, ½ cup raspberries, ¼ high fiber cereal; smoothie (1/2 cup yogurt, 1/2cup skim milk and 1 cup fruit); 1low fat snack bar, 1 apple; ¼ cup raisins, 1 rice cake; 1 orange, 3 cups light microwave popcorn

Exercise Program – Choose one daily - 30 to 60 Minutes Daily - Power Walking, include hills; Break walks into 10 minute intervals if necessary; Cycling, Aerobics Class/Tape, Yoga, Pilates; routines can be split between the morning and evening, i.e., 30 minutes in morning and 30 minutes in evening
15 Minutes toning 4 times per week (Resistance Band, Circuit Training, Free Weights)

Chapter 10
Support Groups

Remember to pray, meditate, and journal your food and feelings. Ask God for everything, and believe that you shall receive it. The house you live in is the house YOU live in! Make it as beautiful on the inside as it is on the outside. Check out http://www.hw.empowerus.net and let us know how you are doing. Join a support group, or start/join a walking club! Health & Wellness kits are available to supplement this book too!

Contact http://www.hw.empowerus.net for more information. Make this a life-long change! Do it for yourself today! Maintenance equals healthy living! Laugh, live, and love!

Starting a support group is easy. Contact like-minded friends who will commit to meet once per week to provide tips, encouragement, and love. You can accept donations to support any materials or healthy snacks the group may want to include in the meetings. Donations can also be for a cause that the group may want to support. If you want to join an existing group find one where donations are accepted, but no fee is required. The internet has a plethora of information that can assist in your lifestyle change.

If you look at the maintenance menu plans, you will see that you can eat what your family eats to a certain degree. You have to drink lots of water and pray profusely. You may fall short, but at least you will be on a path to healthy living on the inside that will be present on the outside, too.

Contact us for more information on how support groups can help. Remember, whatever group you join or start, God should be in the center. This is going to work only if you are committed.

What you have to do is follow the instructions to the best of your ability and continue to build a relationship with God without excuses. I have added Romans 7 in the summary to show that the Bible says that we continue to fall short, but God loves us anyway. Jesus died for our sins precisely because we are going to fall short.

Trust in the Lord and He shall give you the desires of your heart. *Psalm 37:4*

Chapter 11
Summary

I can anticipate the response that is coming:
"I know that all God's commands are spiritual,
but I'm not. Isn't this also your experience?"
Yes. I'm full of myself—after all, I've spent a
long time in sin's prison. What I don't
understand about myself is that I decide one
way, but then I act another, doing things I
absolutely despise. So if I can't be trusted to
figure out what is best for myself and then do
it, it becomes obvious that God's command is
necessary.

But I need something more! For if I know the
law but still can't keep it, and if the power of
sin within me keeps sabotaging my best
intentions, I obviously need help! I realize that
I don't have what it takes. I can will it, but I
can't do it. I decide to do good, but I don't
really do it; I decide not to do bad, but then
I do it anyway. My decisions, such as they
are, don't result in actions. Something has
gone wrong deep within me and gets the better
of me every time.

It happens so regularly that it's predictable.
The moment I decide to do good, sin is there
to trip me up. I truly delight in God's

commands, but it's pretty obvious that not all of me joins in that delight. Parts of me covertly rebel, and just when I least expect it, they take charge.

I've tried everything and nothing helps. I'm at the end of my rope. Is there no one who can do anything for me? Isn't that the real question?

The answer, thank God, is that Jesus Christ can and does. He acted to set things right in this life of contradictions where I want to serve God with all my heart and mind, but am pulled by the influence of sin to do something totally different. *Romans 7:14-25*

God Bless You!

Melanie Denise Magruder

WHAT ABOUT GOD?

Healthy Weight Loss
Through
Commitment, Meditation, & Prayer!

- Weight loss eating plans
- Journal
- Bible Verses
- And more . . .

Bibles Used:

The Message Remix
Aramaic Bible
Women's Recovery Bible
King James Version

PERSONAL NOTES:

PERSONAL NOTES:

PERSONAL NOTES:

PERSONAL NOTES:

PERSONAL NOTES:

PERSONAL NOTES:

PERSONAL NOTES:

PERSONAL NOTES:

PERSONAL NOTES:

PERSONAL NOTES:

PERSONAL NOTES:

PERSONAL NOTES:

PERSONAL NOTES:

PERSONAL NOTES:

PERSONAL NOTES:

PERSONAL NOTES:

PERSONAL NOTES:

PERSONAL NOTES: